Table of Contents

Executive Summary

Governance

Achievement of comprehensive, effective domestic and international biosurveillance is compromised by jurisdictional complexity and inefficiencies. Federal biosurveillance policy oversight should be established in the Executive Office of the President (EOP) with the National Security Staff (NSS) as the lead entity identified to coordinate investments, interagency collaboration, and program implementation including those activities in support of the President's Global Health Initiative. An outside representative advisory group should be established to facilitate key stakeholders' interface with White House policy and technology coordinating groups.

Information Exchange

Methods and metrics used in acquiring biosurveillance data are highly variable. This impedes data sharing and analysis, and recognition and response to health threats. Efficient, comprehensive aggregation and analysis of actionable biosurveillance data should be promoted through support for implementation of IHR 2005; integration of human, animal, food, vector, and environmental surveillance systems into a national biosurveillance strategy; and expansion of biosurveillance to include environmental aspects that are the greatest threat to human health, including water, food, animals, and vectors.

Workforce

The current biosurveillance workforce is inadequate to address existing challenges to biosecurity let alone those that are anticipated to arise with increasing data, globalization, and synthetic biology. The federal government should promote and ensure a sustainable interdisciplinary workforce with investments in expertise, especially in public health informatics; social and behavioral epidemiology; environmental, human and animal health; vector biology; and disaster response.

Research and Development

The federal government should continue to invest in a new generation of research to develop and build on innovative technologies in molecular and cellular sciences, engineering, chemistry, physics, information technology, mathematics, and communications that will enhance the efficiency and sensitivity of regional, national and global biosurveillance. Understanding the baseline and variance of human and animal health using these emerging technologies with clear processes to select the best approaches and scale them will allow for the creation of the functional equivalent of a national and international immune system that can protect the public in real time.

NBAS Membership List

Co-Chairs

Jeffrey P. Engel, MD
State Health Director
Division of Public Health,
Raleigh, NC

W. Ian Lipkin, MD
John Snow Professor of Epidemiology
Professor of Neurology and Pathology
Director, Center for Infection and Immunity
Mailman School of Public Health and
College of Physicians and Surgeons
Columbia University
New York, NY

Designated Federal Official

Pamela S. Diaz, MD
Director, Biosurveillance Coordination
Public Health Surveillance Program Office,
OSELS
Centers for Disease Control and Prevention
Atlanta, GA

Steering Committee Members

Don Burke, MD
Dean, Graduate School of Public Health
University of Pittsburgh
Pittsburgh, PA

Steven H. Hinrichs, MD
Chair, Department of Pathology and Microbiology
College of Medicine
University of Nebraska Medical Center
Omaha, NE

Robert P. Kadlec, MD
Vice President PRTM Management Consultants LLC
Washington, DC

James (Jamie) Allen Heywood
Chairman and Co-Founder
PatientsLikeMe, Inc.
Cambridge, MA

James M. Hughes, MD
Professor of Medicine and Public Health
Emory University
Atlanta, GA

Lonnie King, DVM
Dean, College of Veterinary Medicine
Ohio State University
Columbus, OH

Members

Tomas Aragon, MD, DrPH
Principal Investigator and Executive Director
Center for Infectious Disease & Emergency
Readiness
UC Berkeley School of Public Health
Berkeley, CA

Alvin C. Bronstein MD, FACEP
Associate Professor
Department of Clinical Pharmacology and
Emergency Medicine
University of Colorado Denver, School of Medicine
Medical Director Rocky Mountain Poison Center
Denver, CO

Rita R. Colwell, PhD
Senior Advisor and Chairman Emeritus
Cannon U. S. Life Services, Inc.
Distinguished Professor, University of Maryland
College Park, MD

Julia E. Gunn, RN, MPH
Director, Communicable Disease Control Division
Infectious Disease Bureau
Boston Public Health Commission
Boston, MA

Tom Inglesby, MD
Chief Executive Officer and Director
The Center for Biosecurity of UPMC
Baltimore, MA

Ann Marie Kimball, MD, MPH, BS
Director, APEC EINet
Professor of Epidemiology
University of Washington
Seattle, WA

James W. LeDuc, PhD
Professor, Microbiology and Immunology
Robert E. Shope M.D. and John S. Dunn
Distinguished Chair in Global Health
Director, Galveston National Laboratory
University of Texas Medical Branch
Galveston, TX

Kenneth D. Mandl, MD, MPH

Lawrence (Larry) Brilliant, MD, MPH
President
Skoll Global Threats Fund
Palo Alto

Heather Case, DVM, MPH, Dipl. ACVPM
Director, Scientific Activities Division
Coordinator, Emergency Preparedness and
Response
American Veterinary Medical Association
Schaumburg, IL

David R. Franz, DVM, PhD
VP and Chief Biologial Scientist
Midwest Research Institute
Frederick, MD

James (Jim) L. Hadler, MD, MPH   (Retired)
Former State Epidemiologist and Former Director,
Infectious Diseases Section
Connecticut Department of Public Health
New Haven, CT

Paul E. Jarris, MD, MBA
Executive Director
Association of State and Territorial Health Officials
Arlington, VA

Marcelle C. Layton, MD
Assistant Commissioner
Bureau of Communicable Disease
New York City Department of Health and Mental
Hygiene
New York, NY

Cecil O. Lynch, MD, MS
Assistant Professor
Department of Pathology
University of California at Davis
Granite Bay, CA

Linda A. McCauley, PhD, RN, FAAN

Associate Professor, Harvard Medical School and
Director, Intelligent Health Laboratory,
Children's Hospital Informatics Program
Children's Hospital Boston
Boston, Massachusetts

Kathleen Miner, PhD, MPH, CHES
Associate Dean, Applied Public Health
Emory University School of Public Health
Atlanta, GA

Richard Platt, MD, MSc
Professor and Chair, Dept of Population Medicine,
Harvard Medical School and Harvard Pilgrim
Health Care Institute; Executive Director, Harvard
Pilgrim Health Care Institute
Boston, MA

Thomas R. Slezak, MS
Associate Program Leader, Informatics
Lawrence Livermore National Lab
Livermore, CA

Mary Elizabeth Wilson, MD
Associate Professor of Global Health and
Population
Harvard School of Public Health
Washington, DC

Dean of Nursing
Nell Hodgson Woodruff School of Nursing
Emory University
Atlanta, GA

Stephen M. Ostroff, MD
Director, Bureau of Epidemiology
Pennsylvania Department of Health
Harrisburg, PA

Arthur L. Reingold, MD
Professor and Division Head
Division of Epidemiology
University of California, Berkeley
School of Public Health
Berkeley, CA

Perry F. Smith, MD
Director, Division of Epidemiology (Retired)
New York State Department of Health
Albany, NY

Acronym Glossary

Acronym	Expansion
ACD	Advisory Committee of the Director
APEC EINet	Asia Pacific Economic Cooperation Emerging Infections Network
APHA	American Public Health Association
APHL	Association of Public Health Laboratories
ASM	American Society for Microbiology
ASTHO	Association of State and Territorial Health Officials
ASTM	American Society for Testing and Materials
AVIA	American Veterinary Medical Association
AVMA	American Veterinary Medical Association
BIWAC	Biosurveillance Indications and Warning Analytic Community
BSE	Bovine Spongiform Encephalopathy
CCD	Continuity of Care Document
CCR	Continuity of Care Record
COMTRADE	International Commodities Trade Dataset
CSTE	Council of State and Territorial Epidemiologists
CTSI	Clinical and Translational Science Institute
DARPA	Defense Advanced Research Projects Agency
DHB	Defense Health Board
DMAT	Disaster Medical Assistant Teams
DOD	Department of Defense
DSA	Data Sharing Agreements
EHR	Electronic Health Records
EOP	Executive Office of the President
EPA	Environmental Protection Agency
ePCR	electronic Patient Care Record
EPT	Emerging Pandemic Threats
ER	Emergency Room
FAO	Food and Agriculture Organization
FAOSTATS	Food and Agriculture Organization, Statistics Division
FDA	Food and Drug Administration
GDD	Global Disease Detection (CDC)
GHI	Global Health Initiative
GOARN	Global Outbreak and Alert and Response Network
HHS	Department of Health and Human Services
HIE	Health Information Exchange
HIPAA	Health Insurance Portability and Accountability Act

Acronym	Expansion
HITECH	Health Information Technology for Economic and Clinical Health Act
HL7	Health Level Seven
HSPD-21	Homeland Security Presidential Directive – 21 (Public Health and Medical Preparedness)
IATA	International Air Transport Association
ICSR	Individual Case Safety Report
IHR	International Health Regulations
IOM	Institute of Medicine
ISDS	International Society for Disease Surveillance
LAG	Lead Advisory Group
MMWR	Morbidity and Mortality Weekly Report
NACCHO	National Association of County and City Health Officials
NBAS	National Biosurveillance Advisory Subcommittee
NBSB	National Biodefense Science Board
NEMSIS	National EMS Information System
NGA	National Governors Association
NGO	Non-Governmental Organization
NIH	National Institutes of Health
NSC	National Security Council
NSS	National Security Staff
OIE	World Organization for Animal Health
OMB	Office of Management and Budget
OSELS	Office of Surveillance, Epidemiology, and Laboratory Services
OSTP	Office of Science and Technology Policy
PH	Public Health
PHI	Public Health Informatics
PHII	Public Health Informatics Institute
PHIN	Public Health Information Network
PTSD	Post Traumatic Stress Disorder
R&D	Research and Development
SARS	Severe Acute Respiratory Syndrome
TB	Tuberculosis
USAID	United States Agency for International Development
USDA	United States Department of Agriculture
USG	United States Government
USGS	United States Geological Survey
VA	United States Department of Veterans Affairs
WHO	World Health Organization

NBAS Recommendations

Background

In 2007, Homeland Security Presidential Directive 21 "Public Health and Medical Preparedness" (HSPD-21) was issued in recognition of the emergence of health-related security threats to the nation. Among the mandates in HSPD-21 was the establishment of a federal advisory committee that includes "representatives from state and local government public health authorities and appropriate private sector health care entities, in order to ensure that the federal government is meeting the goal of enabling State and local government public health surveillance capabilities." The federal Department of Health and Human Services (HHS) was charged with this mandate and delegated its implementation to the Centers for Disease Control and Prevention (CDC). On May 1, 2008, the CDC established the National Biosurveillance Advisory Subcommittee (NBAS) comprising prominent experts from the public health, health-care delivery, academic, homeland security, defense and private sectors to provide counsel to the federal government through the Advisory Committee of the Director (ACD) regarding the broad range of issues impacting the development and implementation of a nationwide biosurveillance strategy for human health. The first report, "Improving the Nation's Ability to Detect and Respond to 21st Century Urgent Health Threats: First Report of the National Biosurveillance Advisory Subcommittee" was released on October 16, 2009. Five major recommendations were made to ensure and continue building an adequate biosurveillance capacity for the nation. These included:

- The Executive Branch must define the strategic goals and priorities of federal investments in biosurveillance activities and technologies, and implement a plan to achieve, fund and periodically assess progress toward these goals. To accomplish this, the White House should establish an Interagency Biosurveillance Coordination Committee.

- The U.S. National Biosurveillance Enterprise must include global health threats in its purview and scope.

- The federal government must make a sustained commitment toward ensuring adequate funding to hire and retain highly competent personnel to run biosurveillance programs at all levels of government.

- Government investments in electronic health records and electronic laboratory data should be leveraged to improve how they serve biosurveillance and public health missions.

- The federal government must make strategic investments in new technologies (e.g., genomics, supply chain management, visualizations, display dashboards) to strengthen U.S. biosurveillance capabilities.

Of particular importance, it was noted that much of the domestic biosurveillance workforce capacity to detect, investigate, monitor and respond to public health events is located in state and local health departments, that this capacity has been built with federal public health funding and is in jeopardy with decreasing federal investment in preparedness. Since the first report, these recommendations have not been fully implemented. However, the NBAS-2 recognizes their importance and continued relevance to maintaining and building on current capacity, particularly in the current economic situation with decreasing state and local investment in biosurveillance. This second report reflects the research and deliberations of a newly constituted NBAS established in the spring of 2010 (NBAS-2). Recommendations of the NBAS-2 build on those of the NBAS-1 and differ chiefly in emphasis on prioritization of areas for investment that reflect lessons learned from the H1N1 influenza pandemic, the rise of synthetic biology, and challenges of an austere economic environment.

Biosurveillance refers to the collection, management and integration of health-related data for the purpose of improving detection, characterization, prevention and management of health hazards. This report summarizes current NBAS concerns and challenges regarding governance; collection, exchange, and analysis of health information; and workforce needs. It also provides specific recommendations designed to enable rigorous, comprehensive, and efficient biosurveillance through modifications in governance, standardization of data collection, and investments in informatics, workforce education, and research and development (R&D) across geographic and thematic borders.

Governance

Comprehensive, efficient biosurveillance requires coordination among the public (local, state, and federal) and private sectors. Many institutions critical to biosurveillance operate under their own standards and practices. Moreover, despite increasing availability of electronic health records (for both humans and animals), standardized methods for collecting, analyzing, and sharing public health-related information across the private sector and local, state and federal agencies are lacking, hampering effective integration across jurisdictions. The inadequate information flow across agencies results in federal health-related policies that lack valuable insight and potential guidance from the private sector and state and local agencies. It also diminishes the probability of the functional effectiveness of early detection and response to health threats.

The NBAS reiterates an earlier recommendation that the federal government vest a lead entity in the White House the authority and responsibility for coordinating integration, collaboration, and cooperation among federal agencies conducting biosurveillance activities and to promote public, private, and state and local government agencies involved in biosurveillance. At present, the NBAS is the only federal advisory board capable of providing expert advice to that lead entity on human health-related biosurveillance only. However, the scope of its expertise should be expanded to include food safety, animal and environmental health if it is to serve as the nation's leading biosurveillance advisory committee.

This lead entity should identify strengths and gaps in biosurveillance; mandate development of standardized methods for evaluating and measuring outcomes; support international development of sustainable biosurveillance capacity; integrate plant, animal, relevant environmental and human health information; and supervise the creation of a public database cataloging biosurveillance efforts. It should also enhance communication, and reduce potential for inter-agency duplication of effort and conflict. Biosurveillance efforts must be global in scope and enable early detection and response to health threats.

Challenges

- Requirements for global, borderless biosurveillance: Biosurveillance efforts must be domestic and international in scope, because health threats that emerge anywhere may cross borders quickly and threaten people worldwide.
- Complicated Jurisdictional Oversight: Ideally, a governance structure at the Executive Office of the President is needed to oversee biosurveillance programs across the federal agencies to align efforts, prevent duplication, eliminate inefficiencies, resolve conflicts and promote effective communication and information sharing.
- Obligations under the International Health Regulations (IHR): The 2005 revision to the IHR notes specific activities designed to ensure that every country has the capacity to conduct disease surveillance, and to identify, report, and respond to health events. The IHR represents the most effective mechanism to channel investments to build worldwide biosurveillance capacity.
- Maximizing Private/Public Partnerships: White House policy oversight should promote coordinated national biosurveillance activities that ensure input from the federal, state, and local public and private sectors. U.S. contributions to global disease detection are also dependent on improved/coordinated interactions with public-private partnerships, including but not limited to international, federal, and local agencies; professional societies; businesses; academic institutions; healthcare entities; and non-governmental organizations.
- Issues concerning access: Actors in the public and private sectors may be reluctant to exchange information without explicit assurance that it will not be released to others without permission.
- Inequalities pertaining to data ownership vs. use: There are significant disparities between the federal and the local levels in terms of ownership and need for/use of data; coordination of public health data needs to include all levels.
- Siloed Data: Fractured information flow, due to incompatible surveillance systems, limits the public health system's ability to monitor and improve the delivery of interventions. Public health surveillance programs that develop in silos without attention to inter-operability tend to collect data that are difficult to integrate.

Recommendations

- Establish a robust mechanism for federal policy oversight and coordination, through the Executive Office of the President with the National Security Staff as the lead entity for USG domestic and international (global) biosurveillance programs and activities.

- o Ensure input from federal, state, local and private biosurveillance entities.
- o Align and prioritize Department, Agency and private sector strategies to capitalize on potential synergies and opportunities for improvement.
- o Identify opportunities for improvement based on reviews of recent national and international events such as the H1N1 influenza pandemic, the H5N1 epizootic, Hurricane Katrina and the Deep Water Horizon Disaster.

- Create collaborative mechanisms whereby stakeholder public health and non-governmental organizations, designated representatives of existing federal biosurveillance-related advisory groups, as well as other representative private sector entities, can interface with the White House policy and technology coordinating groups.
  - o Establish a lead advisory group (LAG) composed of representatives from state and local public health and relevant NGOs (ASTHO, NACCHO, CSTE, APHL, NGA) and federal biosurveillance advisory groups (e.g. NBAS, NBSB and designated private entities - a partial list includes agriculture, plant and crop sector, pharmaceutical industry, retail pharmacies, and healthcare organizations and institutions).
  - o The LAG should participate in periodic performance assessments of ongoing domestic and international biosurveillance activities that reflect actual events, exercises and simulations.
- The federal government should identify a single lead entity with responsibility, authority, and accountability to coordinate investments, ensure interagency collaboration and cooperation, and demand efficiency in program implementation of biosurveillance activities supporting the President's Global Health Initiative (GHI).
  - o Develop and maintain a process to inventory and document current and planned investments across the full spectrum of activities relevant to biosurveillance that includes all US government agencies and programs (such as DOD overseas labs, HHS, Global Disease Detection [GDD] Centers [CDC], and the Clinical Trials Network [NIH]).
  - o Consolidate US government investments among agencies and leverage partner agencies and organizations, NGOs, foundations, the business sector, and civil society in host nations, to ensure efficiency, avoid conflict, and maximize return on investment.
  - o Establish metrics for monitoring implementation and outcomes.
  - o Ensure that programs and activities are recognized by host nations and regional partners as aligned with country infectious disease priorities.
  - o Advocate for an international legal framework that coordinates and prioritizes animal health programs.

Information Exchange

Efficient, comprehensive aggregation and analysis of actionable biosurveillance data is compromised by the lack of common descriptors and methods for collection of information as well as inadequate data sharing and use agreements. Standards, metrics, validation protocols, diagnostic platforms, terminology, operational systems, and cultures vary by region, making it difficult for different agencies to seamlessly share information. Additional impediments include intellectual property and indemnity concerns, as well as jurisdictional issues that preclude sharing samples and data. Moreover, the nation's current biosurveillance initiative lacks an integrated surveillance system that monitors the interaction between agricultural, environmental, animal, and human health-related issues. This information gap further hinders surveillance, analysis, and timeliness.

It is imperative that the federal government develop operating principles for data collection, integration, and sharing that allow for flexibility, expansion and innovation. These principles must promote IHR implementation and competencies domestically across states and abroad in partnership with the WHO and regional agencies, ensuring that data is shared among relevant stakeholders, and encouraging cooperation at local, regional, and federal levels. Most importantly, it must create an inclusive biosurveillance system capable of monitoring and integrating environmental, agricultural, animal, and health-related data.

These goals can be accomplished through the adoption of standard protocols, validation and use of broadly applicable metrics based on quantitative research, development of technologies that facilitate real-time data collection, reporting, and analysis, creation of nominal and computation models of disease and wellness, and use of digital clinical records. The federal government should also experiment with leveraging public media and other non-traditional data sets (social networks, user-sourced information, podcasts, and search engine queries) to collect and disseminate information, gain novel insights into population health trends, detect anomalies in health behavior and healthcare consumption, and organize stakeholders who support and promote biosurveillance efforts.

Challenges

- One Health: Domestic animal, wildlife and plant disease surveillance systems and food and vector disease monitoring systems should be integrated into the national biosurveillance strategy for human health.
- Normalized data and Interoperability: The biosurveillance enterprise requires data sharing, systems integration, efficient and timely exchanges of information, standardized diagnostic platforms, interoperable information technologies, and broad data access.
- Common Standards: Metrics must be established to assess the utility of tools, training programs and strategies employed to support national and global biosurveillance efforts.

- Data Use Agreements: Data sharing agreements are an essential building block for developing national and international capabilities, addressing concerns of trust, responsibility, and liability.
- Jurisdiction: Electronic health data are increasingly available. Biosurveillance is dependent upon transmission of these data across jurisdictional lines.
- Language: Variability in terminology is a barrier to biosurveillance. Standardization of methods for recording and reporting information is critical to realizing the promise of data sharing, informing biosurveillance and facilitating situational awareness and event detection.
- Data Sharing: Proprietary diagnostic and disease data from animal and wildlife populations should be shared with public health officials; issues of incentives, confidentiality, and potential political and economic consequences must both be understood and overcome.

Recommendations

- Establish a legal framework for data sharing between state and federal agencies to facilitate information exchange at the state and federal levels.
- Support implementation of IHR 2005:
    - US efforts to support IHR implementation should be conducted in close cooperation with the WHO and its regional affiliates.
    - Communication and coordination with WHO should be enhanced by secundment of an individual from CDC to the IHR implementation unit at WHO.
    - The US should promote IHR implementation using various bilateral, multilateral, and regional diplomatic and security initiatives and encourage other countries to prioritize IHR implementation.
    - Programs should contain objective outcome measures by which progress in building global biosurveillance capacity can be assessed and the benefits of these investments should be documented.
    - The US should objectively target resources toward countries and regions that need additional support to develop capacity to conduct surveillance and response activities as required by the IHRs.

- Integrate domestic animal, wildlife, plant, food, vector, disease and environmental surveillance systems into a national biosurveillance strategy for human health.
    - The USDA, CDC, EPA, USGS, and FDA should work in concert with state agriculture and public health agencies; animal health diagnostic, private food and animal health laboratories; poison centers and their National Poison Data System (NPDS) to collect and analyze surveillance data. These data should be shared with the OIE, FAO, and WHO when appropriate.

- Expand biosurveillance to include environmental sites of greatest threat to human health.

- Biosurveillance should incorporate more microbial and chemical testing, and emphasize recreational and drinking water sites and systems.
- Biosurveillance should consider low level exposures that, over time, may result in human hazards and chronic illness and conditions.
- State and local environmental protection organizations and private corporations should be recruited to ensure access to local expertise.

Workforce

The success of a coordinated biosurveillance system relies on the development of a sustainable interdisciplinary workforce with expertise in disciplines classically associated with public health such as epidemiology, microbiology and other laboratory-based sciences, biostatistics and management but also in others including but not limited to medical and bioinformatics, mathematics, information technology and computer engineering. The NBAS specifically noted a dearth of expertise in social, behavioral, and mental health epidemiology, vector biology, environmental studies, and public health informatics. Social and behavioral epidemiology have the potential to minimize morbidity and mortality and economic costs and improve community resiliency associated with a wide range of acute and chronic disorders. A new medical, public health and bioinformatics workforce will be needed to manage and analyze the exponential increase in volumes of data collected through enhanced biosurveillance efforts. The federal government, in collaboration with domestic and international public and private institutions, should invest in masters, doctoral, and continuing education programs that support the development of personnel infrastructure to address these needs. It should also promote collaboration among basic science, clinical, and public health professionals and ensure strategic placement of individuals with complementary expertise so as to maximize benefits and minimize redundancy and inefficiencies. The NBAS believes that vicissitudes in funding, particularly at the state and local levels, have been an impediment to the recruitment of creative, dedicated individuals to public health. Thus, a commitment to ongoing support will be key to sustainable biosurveillance.

Challenges

- Interdisciplinary capacity: Individuals with a wide variety of skills are needed to support biosurveillance, particularly in informatics, vector biology, behavioral epidemiology and environmental health.
- Training programs: Training programs are currently insufficient to develop the personnel infrastructure for the biosurveillance mission.
- Sustainability: Recruiting and retaining biosurveillance professionals requires a sustained funding commitment.

Recommendations

- Enhance the public health informatics, social and behavioral epidemiology, vector biology and environmental health professions.
  - Support the development and continuity of masters, doctoral and fellowship programs.

- Develop the science of public health informatics through extramural grant research programs.
  - Provide a tuition support program for state and local PH professionals and define and support sustainable biosurveillance career paths.

- Integrate the human and animal health professions
  - Encourage cross training and collaboration of clinicians and basic scientists in human and animal health.

Research and Development

The federal government should invest in research to develop and build on innovative technologies in molecular and cellular sciences, informatics, engineering, chemistry, physics, mathematics and communications that will enhance the efficiency and sensitivity of regional, national and global biosurveillance. The first NBAS report described a DARPA model for identifying initiatives with potential to support this objective. Key impediments to implementing new technologies are the lack of baseline data on biomarkers for individual and population health and disease, samples for assay optimization and validation, and the timeline and expense of pursuing regulatory compliance. Broadly applicable metrics based on quantitative research must be developed, validated, and adopted across agencies using standardized practices. Clinicians, public health professionals, and investigators must collaborate to develop and implement diagnostic and discovery platforms for use in clinical and environmental surveillance. The federal government should encourage data sharing and analysis across jurisdictions, invest in models that track population health across geographic and thematic borders, and leverage data obtained through crowd-sourcing and social networks.

Challenges
- Incentivizing Innovation: Many innovative efforts in data/information mining originate in the private sector. Incentives and funding will be critical to focusing these efforts on biosurveillance.
- Leverage Social Media: Data streams associated with social media or crowd-sourced knowledge have potential to provide new and early insights into population health.
- Aggregation and Analysis of Various Data Sources: The need for data integration, communication networking, and situation awareness has become more acute with globalization and the increasing availability and complexity of health-related information. Methods must be established to rapidly, reliably, and securely collect, synthesize, and share biosurveillance information amongst stakeholders.
- Streamlined Process for Developing/Validating Tools: Currently there is limited process clarity for validating and introducing improved tools or biosurveillance assays. This stifles innovation,

reduces quality and increases costs. There is a need to formalize processes for developing, validating, and deploying tools needed for biosurveillance.

- Diagnostics: Technical innovations based on molecular techniques are increasing the specificity, speed, reliability, and availability of diagnostic testing. There is need for fast, reliable, specific, point-of-care diagnostics and standardized electronic reporting of results for early detection of emerging diseases in both animals and humans.
- Modeling: The potential use of models to anticipate the potential spread of disease and identify probable outcomes given options for interventions is under-utilized and under-funded.
- Defining Health: Disease is deviation from equilibrium "healthy" status. An ideal biosurveillance system needs to baseline health so it can detect deviations from health prior to the onset of clinical disease.

Recommendations

- Develop, evaluate and implement new platforms and algorithms for real time data collection and analysis through investments in research and development.
- Develop, evaluate and implement new methods for detection of pathogens, and biomarkers for health, disease, chemical and radiation exposure, and personalized medicine that can be deployed in a variety of settings including low income countries.
- Improve and formalize pathways for assay optimization, validation and implementation by facilitating access to specimens and data, and standardizing and streamlining the process of assay validation and selection across agencies.
- Invest in nominal and computational models richly descriptive of individual health and the behaviors of healthy populations. The tools to conduct point of care assessments of biomarkers or behaviors indicative of disease, once discovered, should be rapidly deployed and stockpiled.

Appendix I:
National Biosurveillance Advisory Subcommittee
Work Group Reports

Governance:

Biosurveillance in the context of human health is the science and practice of managing health-related data and information for early warning of threats and hazards, early detection of events, and rapid characterization of the event so that effective actions can be taken to mitigate adverse health effects.

TF Scope: Governance (Inter-agency Collaboration and Engagement).

There is a need for the creation of a National Biosurveillance Governance Structure that would oversee and coordinate the biosurveillance programs across the federal agencies, and would develop transparent processes for collaboration and coordination that extend across Federal, State, local and private sector biosurveillance activities. Though not formally defined, this National Biosurveillance Enterprise of federal, state, local and private entities requires a mechanism for formal oversight and collaboration. Without such collaboration and oversight, there will be the persistent risk of duplication of efforts, inefficiencies, and problems with communicating surveillance information in standardized formats to facilitate integration and provide situational awareness from a national level. These collaborative and coordinating processes should include a forum to discuss how federal, state, and local public health capabilities and needs can contribute to a global (domestic and international) biosurveillance system by creating common terms of reference and standards, and ensuring that desired activities receive the resources to achieve a sustainable biosurveillance system.

TF Approach

Issue #1: The Federal Government at the White House level has yet to implement a comprehensive mechanism to oversee and coordinate domestic and international US Government (USG) sponsored or funded biosurveillance activities across the federal, state, local and private sector domains.

Discussion

We reiterate the recommendation from the 2009 NBAS report and recommend the establishment of a robust mechanism of White House policy oversight and coordination of USG domestic and USG-funded international (global) biosurveillance activities. We note that since the earlier NBAS report, there are now offices within the National Security Council (NSC) and the Office of Science and Technology Policy (OSTP) that actively provide oversight of some federal biosurveillance activities. This existing oversight should be expanded to create seamless oversight of policy efforts of the National Security Council (NSC) and National Security Staff (NSS). There are already efforts by the NSC to coordinate federal level international biosurveillance activities. There is a need to create a similar domestic policy oversight mechanism within the NSS Resilience Directorate. There also exists an oversight and coordinating group within the OSTP that monitors research and development (R&D) of technology to support biosurveillance programs and activities, but effective overarching policy and R&D oversight is not yet fully defined or functional. In addition, the Office of Management and Budget (OMB) has an essential role to play in this collective oversight. The combined, coordinated efforts by the NSC, NSS, OSTP and OMB could create the kind of comprehensive oversight needed. To date however, their formal connections and relationships have not matured sufficiently to create this desired end-state.

We are optimistic that these White House level offices and efforts will, over time, mature into effective oversight. Until then, however, many Departments and Agencies of the federal government involved in biosurveillance have a variety of committees and advisory groups that provide oversight or guidance. While many Departments and Agencies currently operate under their own strategic plans and processes, a common set of strategic goals or implementation plan aligning or prioritizing their individual efforts does not exist. Without a coherent strategy and implementation plan based on commonly accepted standards and ongoing assessment, there is a risk of redundant or ineffective outcomes or potential gaps and vulnerabilities. In light of current and expected fiscal constraints, such outcomes are particularly worrisome and could jeopardize the achievement and sustainability of a national biosurveillance enterprise. In forging any implementation plan, we would expect that the extensive involvement by the OMB is essential.

The concept of biosurveillance has evolved since the adoption of the Homeland Security Presidential Directive (HSPD) 21 in October 2006. Electronic health data is becoming increasingly available to support biosurveillance efforts, especially with the recent Stage 1 and proposed Stage 2 Meaningful Use criteria from the Health Information Technology Policy Committee under HHS. However, transmission of this data to local and state public health agencies needs to be implemented in a standardized way that will facilitate effective integration across jurisdictional lines. This will require effective governance to ensure the development of data collection, analysis, and integration standards as well as common evaluation plans with input from local, state and federal public health agencies and the health care IT community. Input from state and local public health officials is essential because the authority for and experience with public health surveillance reporting has historically rested with the states. Governance of biosurveillance activities requires state and local public health input, support, and active participation for effective implementation and evaluation.

Recent events such as the 2009-10 H1N1 Influenza Pandemic and the Deep Water Horizon disaster provided new insights and lessons in biosurveillance. We judge that any White House led effort to revise the practice of biosurveillance should include a review of how current systems function in both detecting events of significant public health concern and monitoring the human health impact (i.e., situational awareness), and of revisions of current biosurveillance priorities and funding to help address identified gaps.

Recommendations:

- We recommend that the White House at the level of the Executive Office of the President (NSS, NSC, OSTP and OMB) create a comprehensive oversight mechanism of federal biosurveillance programs and activities.
- The objective of these White House efforts should include coordinated national biosurveillance activities that ensure input from federal, state, local and private biosurveillance entities (See Issue #2).
- This coordination should include aligning existing Department and Agency strategies, plans and programs and prioritizing resources and efforts to capitalize on potential synergies and opportunities for improvement. Identifying opportunities for improvement must involve reviews of recent national events, such as the H1N1 pandemic and the Deep Water Horizon disaster, and ongoing future evaluations of biosurveillance efforts.

Issue #2: Current federal policy and programmatic deliberations and promulgations often suffer from a lack of input from state and local public health authorities and the private sector.

Discussion

Under the current White House oversight of domestic and international biosurveillance, it is very difficult for state and local governmental and private sector entities to provide the kind of insight and input that could assist in creating a seamless, sustainable national biosurveillance system. We recommend creating a collaborative mechanism by which acknowledged federal, state, and local public health and non-governmental organizations (e.g. ASTHO, NACHO, CSTE, APHL, NGA), designated representatives of existing federal biosurveillance-related advisory groups, as well as other private sector entities, could interface with White House policy and technology coordinating groups.

We judge that representatives from these identified groups could provide valuable input, such as:

- Providing descriptions, educating and informing the NSS of current state and local biosurveillance activities
- Identifying opportunities and vulnerabilities
- Recommending improvements
- Providing guidance on prioritizing strategic objectives and actions
- Reviewing and providing feedback on proposed strategy, policy, plans and resource allocations

We recognize that creation of such a group, the Lead Advisory Group (LAG) would have to conform to existing Federal laws and policies. A semi-annual meeting of the LAG with the NSS in a public forum that permits widespread participation an exchange of new ideas, technologies and polices would support this objective.

Recommendations:

- We recommend establishing a LAG, composed of representatives from established state and local public health agencies and relevant NGOs (ASTHO, NACCHO, CSTE, APHL, NGA), chairpersons of the existing federal biosurveillance advisory groups (e.g., NBAS, NBSB, DHB) and designated private entities (TBD).
- This LAG would participate in routine meetings convened by the White House NSC and NSS policy and OSTP technology oversight committees.
- This LAG would also participate in periodic performance assessments of ongoing domestic and international biosurveillance activities that reflect actual events, exercises and simulations.

Issue #3: What is the best future role for NBAS?

Discussion

There are a number of advisory groups that provide directional advice to various agencies and entities about biosurveillance activities affecting human health, including animal, food, agriculture, and environmental factors. For example, the Defense Health Board has a standing subcommittee devoted to disease surveillance activities pertaining to deploying/deployed U.S. forces. The efforts of these groups are often not coordinated.

NBAS is the only group created by Presidential Directive HSPD-21. Under its current charter and configuration, NBAS is dedicated to address only human health biosurveillance issues. We have recommended the creation of a LAG to advise the relevant White House NSC and NSS policy and OSTP technology committees on the diverse disciplines (environmental, agricultural, animal, and human) that comprise a holistic national biosurveillance system. One alternative to creating a new advisory body is to reconfigure NBAS to serve that function.

This approach is consistent with the recommendations contained in the 2009 NBAS report. If it were infeasible to create a LAG to support the policy and programmatic deliberations at the White House level, we would recommend elevating the role and expanding the representation of NBAS. NBAS is the only existing Federal Advisory Board whose specific mandate is to provide expert guidance on biosurveillance pertaining to human health. This is a unique and vital function that resides nowhere else. While the composition of NBAS is not currently optimized to reflect the spectrum of disciplines needed to represent the current breadth of biosurveillance activities, it could be reconfigured to include expertise in the relevant areas of zoonotic diseases, food safety and environmental issues.

Irrespective of its ultimate disposition and mission, we judge that NBAS can best meet its commitments by reporting directly to Director of CDC and ultimately to the White House.

Recommendations:

- NBAS should remain as an advisory group focused on human health surveillance and be changed to report directly to the Director of CDC.
- The NBAS Chairpersons and other designated NBAS members should be statutory members of the LAG.
- If it is not feasible to create a LAG, the NBAS should be reconfigured to perform the function of LAG.

Healthcare and Public Health Information Exchange

Overview and Background of Recommendations

The Healthcare and Public Health Information Exchange Work Group (HPHIE) has identified three broad areas for improvements including: 1. Addressing the Social Context for Health Information Exchange (HIE), 2., Strengthening the Front Lines through HIE, and 3. Achieving the Potential of HIE.

Each of these topics incorporates complex and challenging issues. The workgroup had two objectives:

- Identify high-level recommendations that would significantly improve national capabilities for public health surveillance and response.
- Focus on issues related to acute or large-scale events as well as routine or ongoing health care activities with the perspective that optimal data sharing is necessary to achieve effective biosurveillance.

To accomplish these goals, a general understanding of the obstacles that have prevented greater progress in spite of longstanding agreement that our current capability is not optimal is necessary.

Issue #1: Addressing the Social Context of HIE

If there is general consensus regarding the value of information exchange between Healthcare and Public Health entities, why has it not been achieved? Jurisdictional concerns and questions over who owns samples and data have hindered the implementation of effective HIE.

Disclosure of sensitive information by entities like "Wikileaks" has raised the question of whether the public and responsible officials will accept and participate in the exchange of information when it may be released without permission. To address this point it is necessary to address who owns the data. Currently, public health events are considered local in nature and prevention and intervention take place at the local level. The workgroup endorses this concept; however, it is essential to broaden the perspective and incorporate the federal government to address gaps in functionality. Local jurisdictions miss out on functionality provided by state or federal governments, especially if they do not view collaboration with state and federal agencies as mutually beneficial. These issues are highlighted by friction caused by jurisdictional boundaries. For example, a local epidemiologist may invite the federal government to assist in an investigation only to feel displaced when a team of federal experts arrives, questions the local population, and sends specimens to the CDC. Local officials may also want to understand the scope and source of outbreak before releasing information to other state or federal agencies, thus increasing the potential for further outbreaks. These sensitivities must be addressed in order to achieve effective HIE across jurisdictions. The workgroup believes that if the full benefit of participating in a national system is presented and appropriate safeguards are established, the goal of a national HIE can be achieved.

Issue #2: Strengthening Biosurveillance through HIE

Local health departments and hospitals are on the front lines of health care delivery and public health surveillance and response. In many jurisdictions, first responders (ambulance services, fire departments, paramedics) report to local public health departments. Electronic information exchange has increased the numbers of cases of reportable conditions and events; however, the ability of local jurisdictions to analyze and monitor the data is limited. HIE has the potential to improve detection of and response to public health emergencies. Adoption of electronic health records by local entities varies greatly across the country (see appendix XC.) Electronic health records offer the potential for data mining. The ability of health departments to efficiently manage the influx of information and avoid warehousing data will require standardization of data collection, analysis, and sharing.

Effective response to public health emergencies requires post-event surveillance. Destruction of underlying infrastructure may result in the need for alternative care sites such as Disaster Medical Assistant Teams (DMAT) facilities and on-site clinics at shelters. Post-event surveillance has identified infectious disease outbreaks, increases in carbon monoxide poisoning, and asthma exacerbation post-fires.

Opportunities to improve data collection, monitoring, evaluation and uses during public health emergencies include:

- Developing technologies that facilitate real-time data collection and reporting
- Establishing common metrics
- Simplifying data collection and reporting requirements
- Establishing systems for use routinely and during public health emergencies

Efforts in emergency management informatics include data standardization and messaging, which allow information from the field to inform biosurveillance and provide a more complete understanding of situation awareness and event detection. Ongoing work by DHS and the DOD should be coordinated with the CDC and other public health partners to create a comprehensive biosurveillance system. Coordination of efforts will be essential to maximize the resources at all levels of public health.

Recommendations:

- Coordinate biosurveillance efforts across federal domains.
- Coordination of public health information needs to include federal, state, tribal, regional and local public health departments.
- Support the development of public health infrastructure including analysis, visualization, and decision support.
- Develop a process to define the added value of data from electronic health records and the required tools needed for utility.

Issue #3: Achieving the Potential of HIE

The HPHIE Workgroup identified two broad topics under which specific activities would take place that would accelerate progress:

- Optimizing the data sets and messaging process for HIE
- Improving functional performance through implementation of data sharing agreements

Protecting the health of the American public requires individualized healthcare by the clinical workforce, personal attention to healthy living strategies, and population surveillance by public health authorities. These strategies will enable the detection and amelioration or elimination of threats to the population as a whole.

Although these entities must take some responsibility for a particular segment of healthcare and prevention work, they cannot function independently as there are undeniable requirements for data sharing between these entities. However, the amount of information needed to make health-related decisions across agencies differs widely due to the ways in which health-related data is identified and shared among agencies. These differences in granularity of the information that needs to be shared between entities yields a matrix that will helps us to define a process of "working interoperability" between and across agencies.

The International Society for Disease Surveillance has identified a minimum data set for use in sharing across agencies for effective biosurveillance that includes an electronic healthcare record system and a syndrome surveillance application. The minimum data set is meant to form the baseline requirements for any vendor to meet meaningful use requirements from a public health perspective and to provide working interoperability between vendor applications and any designed surveillance system used to inform aggregate analysis of public health threats. However, it is inadequate for planning and implementing direct interventions based on specific health threats.

This implies that a different set of meaningful use criteria is needed to achieve working interoperability between electronic healthcare applications and local health departments for determining, for instance, an active case of hepatitis C or whether a case of tuberculosis has been treated according to WHO or CDC standards. Different levels of identifier information both from the perspective of patients and health care providers and organizations are needed to achieve public health interoperability. Interoperability must be bidirectional in order to cycle public health knowledge back into clinical settings.

A local public health data exchange requires that the context of the information received be clearly defined and that there be greater privacy protections for these data. This implies a difference in the data use agreements for information shared at this level of granularity than for data shared for syndrome surveillance purposes. This presents not only an information exchange issue, but also a governance issue, with implications for technology implementations.

Given the differences in the granularity of data and the context which must be applied to that data, it is appropriate to think about the different information structures needed to share this data. At the most granular level of information exchange needed for working interoperability between two clinicians caring for an individual patient, a rich context of information must be applied using an appropriate information structure. For electronic healthcare vendors to meet this level of interoperability, the Office of the National Coordinator has prescribed the continuity of care document (CCD) or the ASTM continuity of care record (CCR) as appropriate information structures to transmit data between providers.

The data structure needed to care for individual patients fits much more closely with the requirements of local public health needs than with the current recommendations for meaningful use for public health using the HL7 2.5.1 or 2.3.1 message structures. The FDA has recognized the additional level of granularity required between providers as it looks to solve the problem of adverse event reporting using electronic healthcare records. It is working on the individual case safety report (ICSR), an HL7 Version 3 message enumerating observational elements that are common across the structured document products used in the CCD. These structures provide greater semantic richness of individual datum and also proscribe a rich contextual framework for understanding the data. Providing this richer structure could significantly lessen the burden on public health professionals by promoting better data acquisition.

Recommendations:

- Establish a tiered representation of public health meaningful use data, aligned with its purpose of use and needs of working interoperability at different levels within the public health sector.

Data sharing agreements (DSAs) are an essential building block for developing national capabilities. The Workgroup believes they are one of the most important approaches for addressing key obstacles to achieving uniform HIE. The section on Social Context for HIE has described scenarios related to the specific need for DSAs. To establish the level of trust needed to allow the sharing of information, the provider must know that the transfer will not generate negative outcomes and that all authorities have approved the transfer. Establishing trust requires knowledge of who owns, has access to, and is authorize to determine the distribution of shared data.

A DSA is a legal document or contract in which two or more parties define the conditions and limitations under which data can be shared or exchanged. For purposes of the current recommendation, the goal is to exchange data electronically. The working group has discussed several examples in the private sector related to sharing sensitive information with commercial value and has assembled a non-exhaustive list of existing or time-limited agreements between health care entities (see appendix XZ). DSAs have been put in place during national emergencies; however, it is essential that such agreements be established in the course of routine business. DSAs accelerate information exchange, but such agreements are not in place (with rare exception) between key federal agencies, including the CDC and state and local entities.

The workgroup notes the development of some DSAs between federal agencies; however until the local source of data (state, county, city) is brought into the agreement, these do not achieve long-term HIE goals. The workgroup has considered a number of key issues related to DSA implementation. While a detailed document is beyond the current scope of this report, some general principles have been identified:

- The DSA we are recommending should be considered a "Foundational DSA." It does not limit further development, but rather sets the basis for further expansion depending on need. This foundational approach should incorporate uniform features and should be of value at local, regional, and national levels.
- It should contain generic terms and conditions that could be modified as needed, based on relevant local law and the nature of the data being shared, such as the jurisdiction in which enforceable elements would be determined (State of New Jersey, Federal District Court).

Recommendations:
- OSELS should act as the lead CDC group to implement this proposal.
- Priority should be given to establishing a "Foundational DSA" for state and local public health entities. External PH partners will include ASTHO, CSTE and NACCHO.
- Establish agreements among and between key federal agencies including DHS and DOD. Local partners will want and need to know how broadly the data will be shared because this may determine which agency should generate a follow up contact (i.e. USDA, DHS, FDA).

References.

http://ncb-prepared.org.

MMWR on EMS electronic Patient Care Record (ePCR) data utility:

http://www.cdc.gov/mmwr/preview/mmwrhtml/mm5921a1.htm?s_cid=mm5921a1_e%0d%0a

NHTSA Pan Flu recommendations for EMS Call Centers (See Guiding Principle #4 and Appendix C):

http://www.nhtsa.gov/people/injury/ems/PandemicInfluenza/PDFs/Task%206.1.4.2Lo.pdf

National EMS Information System (NEMSIS)

www.nemsis.org/theProject/whatIsNEMSIShttp://books.nap.edu/openbook.php?record_id=12992&page=63

Work Group Appendix.
XC.

The Health Information Technology for Economic and Clinical Health Act (HITECH) stimulated the adoption of technology to improve patient and population health. The act provides for payments to clinicians and hospitals when they use electronic health records for electronic laboratory reporting, immunizations, and syndromic surveillance. However, there was no funding to support the efforts of public health departments to receive electronic health data. In addition, many local health departments are safety net providers for vulnerable populations. Services provided include primary care, immunizations, and specialty clinical care for conditions such as tuberculosis and sexually transmitted infections. These departments would also be senders of health information. In 2009-2010, 13% of local health departments that provide primary care used a full electronic record.

In 2010, ASTHO conducted a meaningful use readiness assessment of state health departments. As of December 2010, information on readiness was available for 36 states. Only one state was not planning on being prepared to receive reportable laboratory results and immunization information. Of 35 states, 12 (34%) were not planning to be ready to receive HL7 2.5.1, and 11 (30%) were not planning to receive HL7 2.3.1.

#	Question	Currently prepared	Planning to be prepared	Not planning to be prepared	Responses	Mean
1	Reportable Lab Results (for reportable disease information from hospitals)	18	17	1	36	1.53
2	Immunization Information Systems	18	17	1	36	1.53

#	Question				
3	Syndromic Surveillance System	15	8	12	35	1.91

For syndromic surveillance the messaging capacity is as follows:

#	Question	Currently prepared	Planning to be prepared	Not planning to be prepared	Responses	Mean
1	HL7 2.3.1	16	10	11	37	1.86
2	HL7 2.5.1	10	15	12	37	2.05

Appendix XV.

Governance	Information level and structure	Data Sharing Agreement	Identifier levels (most identified level)
Labs/EHR Vendors and their healthcare customers /ISDS/HHS/CDC/DOD/VA	Syndromic data across Federal agencies, various HL7 V2 messages, proprietary formats; data is coarse and high level	Multiple from interagency, hospital, ISDS secondary use to mandated federal in certain reporting cases	De-identified, no linkage needed
CDC/States	CDC Reporting from states, HL7 V2.51 in most cases; various levels of granularity based on Case Definition and program requirements	CDC through CSTE	De-identified, linkage to state identifiers
States/ local health	State Reporting from local health, multiple proprietary formats, some HL7 V2 feeds; intermediate granularity primarily to satisfy case identification requirements (TB an exception in many states)	State law mandate typically	Identified across multiple areas
Local health	Local Health Reporting from clinical providers, mostly paper, proposed HL7 2.5.1; Granular data focused on small subset	State law but also local jurisdictional law	Identified in all cases
Patient/Clinician/FDA	Clinical care data sharing, adverse event reporting Mostly paper or fax mime type based, required to move to CCD and ICSR; Granular data across broad data set	HIPAA, HITECH, FDA, State law requirements	Identified in all cases

Governance reflects the parties involved that request or provide data and have a negotiated agreement on the data shared

Innovative Information Sources:

Topic: Innovations in Biosurveillance

In order to support the NBAS advisory mandate, a working group was established to determine how to leverage innovations to enhance overall capacity to evaluate human health threats. The Innovation Working Group has identified several areas in which near-term investment could strategically advantage long-term public health outcomes:

- Enable multiplex assay development and validation
- Establish and implement methods for characterizing host susceptibility to health threats
- Leverage "crowdsourcing" and social networks to enhance surveillance and public health communication

Issue #1: Assays

The FDA has oversight over approval of diagnostic platforms and assays. FDA approval can take several years, and is done on an *ad* hoc basis, with few published guidelines and benchmarks. In the case of emerging infectious diseases, the process for biomarker discovery, validation, and assay approval and deployment can easily be overcome by events.

Assay validation is not limited to FDA oversight of human clinical diagnostics. Assays for biosurveillance are also overseen by the CDC (e.g., assays used in the nationwide BioWatch Laboratory Response Network), the USDA (agricultural/veterinary assays for plants and animals), the EPA (water safety), and the DOD (assays used by the military for force protection). Each of these agencies has its own validation practices, with little or no coordination between agencies or acceptance of each other's assays as equivalent. Furthermore, despite advances in technologies toward multiplex assays over the past decade, no agency has yet determined how to validate highly multiplexed assays. The validation of synthesized microarrays or genomic sequencing to diagnose pathogens in human, animals, and plants is also lagging far behind the demonstrated research ability for these techniques to provide great advances in health care and biosurveillance in general.

Methods:

Following the initial working group discussion, follow-up interviews were conducted with leading edge stakeholders in assay development, particularly those recognized as "rapidly" innovative. Their best practices were taken into consideration to bolster the committee's recommendations.

Discussion:

The majority of assays for infectious agents are singleplex. Thus, surveillance and differential diagnosis is tedious, and resource-, sample- and time-intensive. Furthermore, singleplex assays may fail completely in the event a new agent emerges. There is no centralized sample or database with which to optimize and validate assays and platforms. Many biomarker assays are initially developed in rodents, but rodents are not good surrogates for human health and disease.

Further, no standard validation procedures exist across agencies to allow mutual acceptance of actionable information from assays used by other agencies. Additionally, validation procedures for highly multiplexed assays, microarrays, or genomic sequencing for clinical diagnostic use are completely lacking.

Recommendations:
- Develop multiplex assays for pathogen detection.
- Integrate data on cellular pathways and biomarkers that can provide insights into host exposure and response.
- Extend research in animal models to nonhuman primates.
- Improve pathways for assay optimization, validation and implementation.

Specific recommendations include:
- Determine "best-in-class" or "gold standard" assays for evaluation of new competitors. These standards should be updated as improvements are developed.

- Development of assay standards for direct versus indirect pathogen detection via host biomarkers and for triage, environmental survey, and human clinical diagnostic assays, as each of these missions has separate cost and sensitivity thresholds.
- Standardization of assay validation and approval process across agencies, including validation procedures for high information content assays (e.g., multiplex PCR, microarrays, next-gen sequencing).

- Improve storage, accessibility, and management of biobanked samples.
- Develop rapid manufacturing capability for reagents of interest.
- Create generic disease discovery assay platforms.

Issue #2: Baselining Human Health
Disease can be defined as a deviation from equilibrium "healthy" status. To better define what should be perceived as "disease," and develop models that can differentiate between well and sick populations we first need to standardize what it means to be healthy.

We conducted a review of existing systems for modeling disease, as well as efforts to generate models of "wellness." Discussions were held with federal stakeholders who innovate in disease monitoring, with reflections on efforts during the H1N1 pandemic.

Discussion:
Biosurveillance is typically conducted through baseline and resampling of human health. Individuals and populations are serially resampled to detect deviations from a standard equilibrium. Measures of health may include but are not limited to death or absentee rates, frequency of ER visits, language usage in search engines, changes in consumer behavior, such as cold medicine purchases, and genomic or proteomic analyses.

Recommendations:

- Further investment should be made in efforts that seek to create nominal and computational models that are richly descriptive of individual health and the behaviors of healthy populations. A variety of emerging modeling techniques can continue to be supported.
- The means to conduct point of care assessments of biomarkers or behaviors indicative of disease, once discovered, must be rapidly deployed and stockpiled in advance of potential pandemics. Emphasis should be placed on improving the accuracy, use, and transparency of methods that do not require direct interaction with patients.

Specific recommendations include:

- Develop passive models that mine "public" or transparent records for disease signatures.
- Validate and verify models of baseline health as well as emerging diseases.

Issue #3: Social Media and Biosurveillance

The biosurveillance enterprise includes a wide range of stakeholders in addition to public health professionals and clinicians. Many of these individuals participate and contribute to social media or crowd-sourced knowledge via Facebook, Twitter, Wikipedia, or similar applications. New and early insights into population health could be realized if these data streams were organized for systematic analysis.

A search was conducted to determine whether a generalized public health online community existed. While disease specific clinical networks do exist, these are generally hierarchical in nature. Additionally, one-off projects based on open platforms such as Google Maps provide an initial view into how information can be managed in such an environment.

Discussion:

Specialized social communities exist in computer programming, are deployed in the intelligence community, and have recently been created to allow sales and marketing specialists to share "leads" between companies. A similar social network would allow for similar value creation in the biosurveillance space. Public social network platforms could be used to create networks of stakeholders who support biosurveillance. Such a network could also exist as a source for passive information collection of public health trends. Questions of credentialing, privacy, and security readily arise in such an environment, and the system would need to balance the quality of information with existing regulatory frameworks such as HIPAA. Tools should be broadly socialized to ensure sustainability.

Recommendations:

- A working group consisting of stakeholders from various agencies and actors in public health should be convened to develop pilot projects in "social media" style platforms.
- Address regulatory, privacy, security and credentialing concerns, data elements of common interest, and tools with immediate utility.

Global and Regional Biosurveillance Collaboration

Introduction

Biosurveillance efforts must be global in scope because health threats that emerge in any part of the world may cross borders and threaten people worldwide. Examples include outbreaks of new, resurgent, drug-resistant, or highly dangerous diseases; pandemics of respiratory diseases like influenza or SARS; and deliberate or accidental release of microbes, chemicals, or radiation into air, water, or food. Mitigation of these dangers requires coordinated and collaborative U.S action that makes optimal use of current tools and opportunities to enhance global disease detection and response.

Scope

The Work Group was charged with exploring ways to more efficiently manage, coordinate, and leverage U.S. government (USG) global health biosurveillance and development policies and activities. The goal is to maximize the effectiveness and impact of the United States' efforts to contribute to and participate in disease detection and response to improve global public health, safety and security.

Approach

The Work Group compiled this report based on the outcomes of two face-to-face meetings, review of dozens of documents stored in Google Docs with open access for all NBAS members, over twenty briefings from multiple agencies, several conference calls, discussions with key stakeholders, and feedback from members on several drafts of the report.

The members of the NBAS Global Workgroup agreed that:

The US has compelling interests in global human and animal health for humanitarian, development, economic, and security reasons.

- Support for the ability of every country to fully implement the International Health Regulations (IHR 2005) is currently the best opportunity for the United States to build global disease detection and response capacity. Assisting individual countries to improve their human and animal biosurveillance capacities benefits their population and other countries around the world, including the U.S.
- Given the adoption of the IHR in 2005 by the World Health Assembly, implementation of these regulations around the world represents a strategic opportunity for the US to advance global health and its own national interests.
- US contributions to and participation in global disease detection and response through an all-hazards approach that increases global capacity and coordinated international action are dependent upon
    - Coordinated, leveraged, and more effectively managed USG bilateral and multilateral global health investments and policies across and within agencies

- Enhanced engagement with WHO, OIE, FAO and other international multi-lateral organizations
- Improved and coordinated interactions with public-private partnerships, professional societies, the business sector, academic institutions, NGOs, and civil society organizations engaged in global public health activities

As part of its deliberations, the NBAS Global Workgroup considered the following issues:

1. Surveillance is the ongoing, systematic collection, analysis and interpretation of data to facilitate timely response. Biosurveillance requires managing health-related data and information for early warning of threats and hazards (both the routine and the unusual), early detection of events, and rapid assessment to facilitate rapid, effective responses to mitigate health effects.
2. Emerging diseases and all other hazards can occur in any location. No country is immune or insulated from these risks, although the types, scope, and vulnerabilities vary from place to place. Therefore, each jurisdiction should have the ability to identify, monitor, and respond to human-, animal-, environmental-, and food-associated public health threats.
3. USG biosurveillance investments are unevenly distributed and are at times driven by strategic and diplomatic priorities rather than public health needs, capacities, and threats and are often short-term and not sustained.
4. In an era of restrained resources, US global investments in biosurveillance must be efficiently managed both centrally and at the country level, avoiding duplication and inefficiencies that result in sub-optimal impact.
5. Non-governmental investments by the philanthropic sector have grown dramatically and are substantially contributing to global biosurveillance. Improved coordination between USG investments, other countries' investments, and these philanthropic efforts would lead to better outcomes and benefits.
6. Capacity within international organizations (e.g., WHO, OIE, FAO) has grown substantially. Providing opportunities to work with and through these organizations to leverage existing U.S. investments would increase their impact.
7. National surveillance capacity, especially within emerging economies, has also increased. These emerging economies can also significantly contribute to improving global biosurveillance.
8. Globally, human public health is intrinsically linked to animal health and agriculture. Biosurveillance investments in these sectors are as strategically important as investments in human health biosurveillance.
9. There is a need for metrics, evaluation, tools and training to monitor and support global biosurveillance efforts.

The NBAS Global Workgroup also identified and considered changes that have taken place over the past 15 years that have modified the environment in which biosurveillance is conducted. The Workgroup identified the following as opportunities upon which to build:

- **U. S. initiatives and investments in global health,** which can be coordinated and synergized for maximum public health impact. Current U.S. initiatives that enhance global biosurveillance include the *National Strategy to Counter Biological Threats*, which promotes global disease detection (http://www.whitehouse.gov/sites/default/files/National_Strategy_for_Countering_BioThreats.pdf); the President's *Global Health Initiative*, which strengthens data collection and diagnostic services in developing countries (http://www.pepfar.gov/documents/organization/136504.pdf); and the USAID Emerging Pandemic Threats (EPT) Initiative which supports global surveillance and response capacity for zoonotic diseases — a major source of emerging threats to human health. US investments in global health include establishment of Global Disease Detection Centers (http://www.cdc.gov/globalhealth/GDD/gddcenters.htm), new Field Epidemiology and Laboratory Training Programs (http://www.cdc.gov/globalhealth/fetp/), and the Global Emerging Infections Surveillance and Response System (http://www.afhsc.mil/geis), among many others.

- **2005 International Health Regulations (**IHR; http://www.who.int/ihr/en/). The IHR provide a legal and political framework for international engagement that ties reporting to response and promotes capacity-building in developing countries. Under the IHR, each WHO member nation must maintain or develop core competencies in disease surveillance, reporting, and response capacity (IHR, Annex 1A), with industrialized nations providing support to developing nations in building and strengthening these competencies (Article 5, IHR). International outbreak assistance is available, if requested, from the Global Outbreak and Alert and Response Network (GOARN; http://www.who.int/csr/outbreaknetwork/en/), which serves as WHO's IHR response arm.

- **Multi-sectoral partnerships,** which can expand and enhance global disease surveillance and response. Biosurveillance partnerships go beyond the traditional healthcare and public health sectors to include animal and environmental health experts (e.g. the One Health Initiative; http://www.onehealthinitiative.com/), trade groups (e.g., Asian-Pacific Economic Cooperation (APEC) EINet; http://depts.washington.edu/einet/about.html), and diplomatic fora (e.g., the Global Health Security Initiative [http://www.ghsi.ca/english/index.asp]), foundations and non-governmental organizations (e.g., the Gates Foundation), multinational corporations, and university research networks.

- **Innovations in telecommunications and molecular diagnostics**, which underpin new methods for data-gathering and laboratory-based biosurveillance. The internet and telecommunications tools have made collection and analysis of large amounts of information operationally feasible— as demonstrated by the Biosurveillance Indications and Warning Analytic Community (BIWAC)— and have helped create global and regional networks that share data on microbial threats. At the same time, technical innovations based on molecular techniques are increasing the specificity, speed, reliability, and availability of diagnostic testing.

Recommendations:

United States Government Leadership

The USG must play a leadership role in coordinating national investments in biosurveillance to ensure optimum return on investment, especially during this era of fiscal austerity, affecting the United States as well as our partners.

1. The USG should identify a single, senior-level lead entity (such as NSS in the EOP) with responsibility, authority, and accountability to coordinate investments, require and ensure interagency collaboration and cooperation, and demand efficiency in implementation of biosurveillance activities in support of the President's Global Health Initiative (GHI).

    - An inventory of current and planned investments across the full spectrum of activities relevant to biosurveillance should be created, along with a process to keep the database up-to-date (i.e., on a quarterly basis). The inventory should contain input from all USG agencies and programs. In addition to surveillance activities, the database should incorporate information on training programs, capacity-building efforts, disease- and pathogen-specific vertical programs, and other relevant activities that could contribute to identification of hazards and improved accuracy, timeliness, and efficiency of USG biosurveillance efforts. The inventory should be easily accessible to all governmental agencies and be publicly available to extra-governmental organizations (e.g., NGOs, private foundations, host nations, and other stakeholders). The inventory should serve as tool to enhance coordination, communication, and efficiency.

    - Investments should be assessed horizontally (across agencies) and on a location-by-location basis to avoid duplication, assure maximal impact, enhance efficiency, and identify priority gaps. When feasible, existing projects with overlapping goals and strategies should be combined, and new projects should be carefully assessed and approved to maximize potential synergies with existing activities and to avoid duplication.

    - USG investments should be consolidated among agencies and leveraged whenever possible with those of partner agencies and organizations, NGOs, foundations, the business sector, host nation civil society, and other stakeholders to ensure efficiency, avoid conflict, and maximize return on investment.

    - Evaluation and outcome measurement must be a key component of each activity and include key metrics indicative of success in achieving specific targets. All investments in biosurveillance must be results-oriented and their impact clearly demonstrated.

    - Sustainability of every global biosurveillance investment must be a key consideration at the onset of any program and be an ongoing consideration during periodic evaluation. Programs and activities must be recognized by host nations and regional partners and aligned with host country infectious disease priorities. Each activity should include a clear exit or transition strategy defined prior to implementation to ensure that the impacts of investments are sustained by the host jurisdiction and region.

Implementation of IHR 2005

The 2005 revision to the IHR contains a specific set of activities designed to assure that each jurisdiction has the capacity to conduct disease surveillance, to promptly identify and report health events that may pose a threat for international spread, and to respond to these threats through timely investigation and implementation of control measures. As a globally agreed upon framework for disease monitoring and control, the IHRs represent the single most effective mechanism to channel investments to build worldwide biosurveillance capacity.

2. Any location can be the source of an emerging global public health threat. Therefore, all jurisdictions need to have systems in place to properly identify, diagnose, investigate, and respond to such threats. IHR implementation at home and abroad is a public health and security priority for the US. The USG should support full and robust implementation of IHR 2005 in every jurisdiction and target and leverage resources to achieve this goal.

   - US efforts to support IHR implementation should be conducted in close cooperation with the WHO and its regional affiliates. WHO is the lead agency for IHR implementation and has created an infrastructure for monitoring and assessing IHR capacity at the country and regional levels. US support for IHR implementation could best be accomplished by working in partnership with WHO to assist specific locations or regions in developing biosurveillance capacity.

   - Communication and coordination with WHO should be enhanced by secundment of an individual from CDC to the IHR implementation unit at WHO.

   - Implementation of the IHR has important security implications for the US, and coordination between DOD and DOS initiatives focused on international threat reduction and disease monitoring programs should be carefully coordinated with other USG partner agencies, WHO, and international partner states and organizations to ensure coordination and cooperation while avoiding duplication of efforts.

   - The USG should promote IHR implementation using various bilateral, multilateral, and regional diplomatic and security initiatives, encourage other countries to prioritize IHR implementation, and support international efforts to increase transparency and sharing of information and etiologic agents that pose potential regional or global threats.

   - Support for IHR implementation is consistent with the priorities of the President's GHI. Programs to build IHR capacity should be developed and implemented within the overall GHI framework.

   - Any programs developed through the GHI process should contain objective outcome measures by which progress in building global biosurveillance capacity can be assessed and the benefits of these investments documented. The US should support development and use of an objective IHR implementation scorecard to measure progress in achieving IHR surveillance goals.

- The US should objectively target resources toward locations and regions that need additional support to develop institutional capacity to conduct surveillance and response activities as required by the IHRs.

- An equivalent framework to the IHR is needed for animal health. The USG should advocate the creation of a similar international legal framework to organize, coordinate, and prioritize animal health biosurveillance emphasizing an all-hazards approach.

Research and Innovation

A robust research agenda to support effective, efficient, and innovative biosurveillance is needed. This research agenda should encompass human, animal, and plant pathogens and diseases; draw on a broad spectrum of approaches and tools including basic biological sciences, ecological approaches, systems research, and social network analysis; build capacity that engages public and private institutions, the business and philanthropic communities, and global partners; and seek to better understand cross-species movement of microbes and the appearance of novel microbes, whether developed through human intent or emerging naturally.

3. The USG should lead the development of a comprehensive research agenda supporting the strengthening of global biosurveillance capacity. Areas of focus should include development and evaluation (sensitivity, specificity, speed, cost, reliability, among others) of new technologies offering the potential for the efficient, effective collection and dissemination of critical information to key individuals:

   - Fast, reliable, specific, point-of-care diagnostics for the early detection of emerging diseases and interruption of their spread (and avoidance of unnecessary interventions).

   - Models used to project "what might happen if" scenarios to anticipate the potential spread of disease and population effects and to monitor how epidemics unfold. These can serve to identify the most likely outcomes given several policy options for interventions.

   - Technologies that can be used for communication, including the use of social networks to report, track, and intervene during outbreaks, and geo-referencing systems that can be used in tracking disease.

   - Capabilities to rapidly recognize emergence of antimicrobial resistance, genetic changes, or recombination events that may lead to more virulent pathogens. Development and validation of metrics for measurement and communication of risk in a way that allows an appropriate level of response. Metrics should be broadly applicable and understandable across many disciplines and based on quantitative or semiquantitative measurements.

- Assessment of the efficacy and effectiveness of research training programs to facilitate adjustments based on findings. Metrics should include sustainability of learned behavior or activity and allow evaluation of effectiveness of different approaches. Feedback on performance should be provided to program leaders so that adjustments can be made when indicated.

- Development of potential climate change scenarios and projections that identify vulnerable places, settings, and populations that may be displaced or otherwise impacted. The scenarios should take into account animal and plant pathogens that have implications for food security.

- Consideration of trade and travel as key factors favoring disease emergence and global spread. To date, the key metrics of interest for these global phenomena have not been identified and systematically evaluated, although global databases are available (e.g., COMTRADE, FAOSTATS, IATA). A research program that tests and incorporates such metrics (i.e., point-to-point connection, load factors for passengers/freight, volume of agricultural commodities, etc.) and rigorously defines their actions on the course of epidemics and pandemics should be implemented. Such systems should be utilized when outbreaks occur to minimize cross-border spread.

Acknowledgements

NBAS Consultants: Ray Arthur, John Ridderhof, Alexandra Levitt

Federal Liaisons: Clifford Brown, Teresa Quitugua, Raul Sotomayor

PHPS/OSELS/CDC Staff: Pamela Diaz, Curtis Weaver, Mark Byers, Danielle Stewart

Emory University Staff: Ashley Freeman

Biosurveillance Workforce & New Professions

Approach

The Task Force began its work in September, 2010 with a series of conference call discussions during which it reviewed the work and recommendations in 2009 of its previous iteration (the NBAS Biosurveillance Workforce of the Future Task Force), defined areas in which it felt additional information was needed, and decided to arrange presentations by key informants involved in workforce development, use of electronic health records for public health surveillance and training of public health informaticians. Following the conference calls and presentations, a face-to-face meeting on January 14, 2011 in Atlanta was held to bring together Task Force members' views of what was most important in this area and to define and develop consensus recommendations on the two or three most important issues relating to its charge.

Endorsement of Previous Recommendations: The Task Force recognized that the previous recommendations were still salient and of critical importance. One of five NBAS final recommendations in 2009 was that "The federal government must make a sustained commitment toward ensuring adequate funding to hire and retain highly competent personnel to run biosurveillance programs at all levels of government."(1) At that time it was noted that federal public health preparedness funding allocated to state and local health departments and schools of public health beginning in 2002 had been critical to building domestic biosurveillance epidemiologic and laboratory capacity for both emergency and non-emergency public health conditions, that the corps of personnel created with it had become the domestic biosurveillance workforce, and that it was critical to maintain rather than allow further erosion of this workforce without at least a thorough assessment of what was needed. Since this recommendation was made, the situation has not improved. No formal assessment has been done; a survey of state health departments by the Council of State and Territorial Epidemiologists in 2009 found that epidemiology capacity for bioterrorism/emergency response peaked in 2006 and has deteriorated since (2,3), most states are reducing their public health workforce in response to the budget crisis that began in September 2008 and in the process have lost but not replaced many experienced leaders, and there are competing public health priorities (e.g., chronic disease, obesity, health disparities) attracting newer leaders. However, the Task Force felt that there were other critically important biosurveillance workforce issues that needed to be and could be addressed independently of the uncertain economic situation and ability to maintain the current workforce. These are the issues the Task Force has chosen to highlight and make new recommendations to address, while acknowledging that the previous workforce-related recommendation still needs critical attention.

New Workforce Requirements in Public health Informatics: Public Health Informatics, defined as the systematic application of information and computer science and technology to public health practice, research, and learning, has become a central function of public health systems and yet this infrastructure is woefully inadequate, fragmented, and underfunded. This fractured information flow limits the public health system's ability to monitor and improve the delivery of interventions for acute or chronic conditions. It causes public health programs to develop in silos and lack coherence with data elements with little or no uniformity. (4) Another important feature of public health's informatics infrastructure is its expected role in collaboration with the larger clinical and response community during a biosurveillance event. The public health system is often the lynch pin of laboratory and other population-based information. (5) In addition to the disarray of informatics systems architecture, the public health workforce does not have sufficient competency-based trainings to work with the pieces of the architecture that may actually be in place within their public health system. For public health systems to achieve their core functions and undertake their charge for biosurveillance, we need a well-trained workforce in the basics of public informatics. In recognition of the desperate need for additional public health informatics capacity both ASTHO and NACCHO have passed policy statements encouraging access training for public health professionals. (6, 7)

During the last decade, public health informatics has become more defined as science and a discipline; some are beginning to call it a profession. This field now has its own competencies and a number of universities are offering degrees and certificates. (8) What this means is that the potential for offering training and/or finding future public health professionals is promising.

Recommendation #1. Strengthen public health informatics as a key element of the future national biosurveillance workforce.

Enhance the public health informatics profession by: 1) developing suitable federal and state job classifications series (e.g. tier I, II, III); 2) increasing the number of formal masters level degree programs in public health informatics; 3) increasing the number of doctoral level degree programs in public health informatics; and, 4) developing the science of public health informatics though extramural grant research programs to study topic such as computational modeling, simulation, decision support, and applications for public health practice.

- Expand the training of the public health workforce by: 1) expanding the public health informatics fellowships programs (e.g. CDC, PHII) in a way that ensures that qualified applicants can be placed to fill the need; 2) developing a public health informatics tuition support program for state and local public health professionals to cover the cost of training in an approved PHI program.; 3) supporting public health informatics professionals to join and or participate in the PHIN, AMIA, and other relevant emerging technology conferences.

- Integrate the public health informatics professionals with other human and animal health professionals by: 1) including social science, mental health, environmental health, and veterinary health professionals in the development public health information systems; 2) encouraging public health informatics professionals within universities to engage with their NIH funded colleagues, notably CTSIs; 3) ensuring that the focus of the public health informative data collection leads to early warning, detection, monitoring, investigation, and inference for the population-based concerns within the community.

New Workforce Requirements in Social, Behavioral and Mental Health: An expected component to any type of disaster or terrorist event is the adverse social or behavioral consequences accompanying the event. In a natural event when human life is threatened and social structures disrupted or destroyed, fear and terror are expected consequences. In the case of terrorist events, the goal of the perpetrators is often not just to inflict death and destruction but also to induce terror throughout the nation. Fear produces stress resulting in mental health casualties. Increased incidence of psychiatric disorders (e.g., generalized anxiety, panic, posttraumatic stress disorder [PTSD], depression), psychological distress (e.g., insomnia, irritability, feelings of vulnerability, work absenteeism, withdrawal, social isolation), and health risk behaviors (e.g., smoking, imbibing alcohol, drug use) can be expected. Numerous studies have documented a heightened prevalence of psychiatric disorders, domestic violence, and substance use in the aftermath of most major disasters (12). Communities impacted by Katrina saw rates of mild to moderate mental illness almost double (10). Rates of mental disorders have also increased in response workers as seen in reports of the impact of the response to the events of September 11, 2001 (8). Social and mental health outcomes were a major area of concern in the consequences of the 2010 Gulf Oil Spill as was also seen during and after similar man-made oil spills throughout the world (11). Analysis of the health consequences of the World Trade Center disaster point out the need for identification of psychological response and at-risk populations that can be targeted for preventive interventions (8). To adequately and rapidly characterize the full scope of the event, integration of surveillance of the mental health or behavioral health consequence is needed. This need was also pointed out in the recommendations of a 2003 IOM report that urged the determination of background rates of behavioral and psychological factors important in predicting psychological consequences. The report pointed out the need for agencies to develop a common protocol and work cooperatively to develop, implement, and sustain comprehensive public health surveillance across phases of a terrorist event.

Effective surveillance and early response to the psychological health impacts of man-made or natural disaster events is compounded by a lack of mental health resources and manpower. Reports focused on the health effects of the 2010 Gulf Oil Spill suggest that mental health was one of the most urgent public health concerns and that while the vast majority of surveillance data collected by the state health offices was for acute physical illnesses public health officers from all five states impacted by the event identified the need for increased and better targeted mental health surveillance as an immediate challenge (11). Historically the social/behavioral workforce has not played an integrated role in biosurveillance events. States' mental health disaster plans have evolved through the years, but they suffer from lack of integrated planning with other health sectors responsible for surveillance and response. In 2003 the U.S. Department of Health and Human Services, Substance Abuse and Mental Health Services Administration, Center for Mental Health Services reported that resources- both human and financial-are key components to successful mental health disaster planning and implementation. Few states, have even a single person whose full-time responsibility is disaster and emergency mental health. (9). Surveillance systems for mental illness and substance abuse must be strengthened with both intellectual and human capital investment. Syndromic surveillance for mental health indicators requires refinement, given the varied somatic manifestations of stress and the potential reluctance of historically marginalized populations to seek mental health or substance-abuse services. Local engagement is key: community agencies can alert public health officials to emerging issues. (12)

Recommendation #2. Enhance the national capacity to assess and manage the psychological dimensions of man-made or natural disasters

- Ensure that social, behavioral and mental health epidemiologists be considered as full members of biosurveillance investigation and monitoring teams, and that when biosurveillance is conducted, it should also focus on indicators of community resiliency.

- Provide training informatics to socio-behavioral and mental health epidemiologists, and recruit social, behavioral and mental health experts into informatics training programs.

References

1. National Biosurveillance Advisory Subcommittee. Improving the nation's ability to detect and respond to the 21st century urgent health threats: first report of the National Biosurveillance Advisory Subcommittee. Report to the Advisory Committee to the Director, CDC, April 2009; pages 1-10. Available at: http://www.cdc.gov/osels/pdf/NBAS%20Report%20-%20Oct%202009.pdf Accessed January 21, 2011.

2. CDC. Assessment of epidemiology capacity in state health departments - United States 2009. *MMWR* 2009; 58(49):1373-1377.

3. CSTE. 2009 National assessment of epidemiologic capacity: findings and recommendations. CSTE 2009. Available at http://www.cste.org/dnn/.

4. Jennifer Ellsworth Fritz, Priya Rajamani, Martin LaVenture (No Date). Developing a Public Health Informatics Profile: A Toolkit for State and Local Health Departments to Assess their Informatics Capacity. The Minnesota Department of Health.

5. Rebecca A Hills, William B. Lober, Ian. S. Painter. (2008). Biosurveillance, Case Reporting, and Decision Support: Public Health Interactions with a Health Information Exchange. BioSecure D. Zeng et al (Eds.) Springer-Verlag: Berlin Heidelberg pps 10-21.

6. NACCHO. (2007). Statement of Policy: Public Health Informatics Workforce (No. 07-06) http://www.naccho.org/advocacy/positions/upload/MicrosoftWord-0706PUBLICHEALTHINFORMATICSWORKFORCE.pdf (retrieved 1/16/2011).

7. ASTHO. (2008). Public Health Informatics Policy Statement. http://www.astho.org/Display/AssetDisplay.aspx?id=165 (retrieved 1/16/3011).

8. CDC. (2009). Competencies for Public Health Informaticians. HHS and the University of Washington Center for Public Informatics. Cone, J. Lessons from the World Trade Center. Presentation to the IOM Committee to Review the Federal Response to the Health Effects Associated with the Gulf of Mexico Oil Spill. September 23, 2010, Tampa, FL.

9. IOM 2003. *Preparing for the Psychological Consequences of Terrorism: A Public Health Strategy.* Washington, DC: The National Academies Press.

10. IOM. 2009. *Assessing Medical Preparedness to Respond to a Terrorist Nuclear Event: Workshop Report*, DC: The National Academies Press.

11. IOM. 2010. *Assessing the Effects of the Gulf of Mexico Oil Spill on Human Health.* Washington, DC: The National Academies Press.

12. U.S. Department of Health and Human Services. *Mental Health All-Hazards Disaster Planning Guidance*. DHHS Pub. No. SMA 3829. Rockville, MD: Center for Mental Health Services, Substance Abuse and Mental Health Services Administration, 2003. Yun, K.Y., Lurie, N., Hyde, P.S. 2010. Moving mental health into the disaster-preparedness spotlight. **New England Journal of Medicine.** 363(13):1193–1195.

Integrated Multi-Sector Information

Task Force Approach

The Task Force on Integrated Multi-Sector Information met on multiple occasions. The Task Force (TF) initially discussed the scope and reach of its work and agreed on a group of subject matter experts to present to the TF and engage in further discussions. The TF reviewed the Concept Plan for Implementation of the National Biosurveillance Strategy for Human Health and the final National Biosurveillance Strategy. The group also reviewed the findings from an earlier NBAS subgroup on "Animals, Food, and Vectors." In addition, the TF reviewed reports from the CDC's Office of Critical Information Integration and Exchange. At a final meeting, the TF synthesized its findings, established priorities, and created five working papers about the Human-Animal Interface; Local State-Global Connectivity; Environmental and Data Base overview; Use of Technology, and Overarching Issues. Finally, these reports were merged into the TF Report and issues and recommendations were finalized from this process.

Introduction

Integrated biosurveillance information was identified as a priority in developing a cohesive strategy for effective national biosurveillance. The objective was to generate actionable health intelligence by increasing access to information resources and synthesizing multiple streams of information into one coherent picture. Key advances in technology, science, and communications need to be leveraged and adapted to achieve effective biosurveillance integration.

There is a critical need to improve and integrate biosurveillance across human and animal health, agricultural, and environmental disciplines to create a One Health model. These domains are inextricably connected. Thus, our ability to identify and respond to hazards impacting human health and to develop an effective national biosurveillance system is dependent on a holistic, integrated strategy that crosses domains, sectors, professions, and data resources. The One Health model emphasizes the need to shift surveillance "upstream" closer to the genesis of the threat to improve prevention, early detection and response.

Specifically, more effective environmental biosurveillance is necessary. Our water sources pose a threat to human health due to microbial and chemical contamination. Disease vectors must be added to an integrated biosurveillance program to improve awareness and track microbial migration prior to human exposure. There is obvious shared responsibility that crosses and includes wildlife, domestic animals, and their products, food, water, environment, and vector monitoring. Data and information sharing must be attained from government agencies, international organizations, poison control centers, food systems, recreational and potable water, and diagnostic labs that are government, university, and private.

Current biosurveillance systems that involve animal, human, and environmental domains, however, are fragmented, with little or no integration. A biosurveillance system that is multi-sectored will need to overcome challenges of information and operational systems that are not standardized or connected;

cultural and incentive differences in sharing data; ensuring integration across agricultural and public health agencies and organizations; and, incorporation of massive amounts of microbial data sets from private and corporate diagnostic labs whose testing results are considered proprietary.

Issue #1

The human-animal interface has progressively increased, creating a greater chance of human exposure to multiple hazards from direct contact with animals or through food and water.

The TF had discussions with USDA and CDC experts in food borne and vector borne illnesses; TF members included representatives from the AVMA and experts in One Health and emerging zoonoses.

Discussions

With the realization that 60% of human pathogens are multi-host microbes, it is abundantly clear that animal populations (domestic, exotic, and wildlife) and their products need to be included in a national biosurveillance plan. The interface between animals and people is both intensifying and accelerating. Today seven billion people share the earth with 25-30 billion food animals, approximately 500 million pets, and countless wildlife and exotic species. Pathogens are transmitted directly from animals or indirectly through food, water, environment, and through vectors such as mosquitoes, fleas, and ticks. These need to be included in a comprehensive biosurveillance strategy.

Accurate and rapid surveillance systems are necessary to detect food-, water-, and vector-borne pathogens. Antimicrobial resistant organisms need to be included in the biosurveillance plan because they are an emerging group of pathogens that may originate in animal species. The global food system needs to be monitored to prevent the transmission of pathogens and to serve as an early warning system. Eighty percent of select agents are zoonotic and may be discovered in animals, animal health diagnostic laboratories or private veterinary clinics before becoming a human threat. Increasing interconnectivity through travel, trade, and new diasporas create unprecedented hazards to human health and represent areas that need to be monitored to achieve early detection and response.

Recommendations:
- Develop a plan to include animal disease surveillance systems (food-animal, exotic, wildlife, and companion) along with food and vector disease monitoring systems, and integrate these into a national biosurveillance strategy for human health.
- The USDA, CDC, and FDA should take responsibility and involve state agriculture and public health agencies, animal health diagnostic laboratories, and private food and animal health laboratories. These agencies should also collaborate with and share surveillance data with the OIE, FAO, and WHO.

Issue #2

There is a critical need to maximize connectivity and utilization. Expansive biosurveillance data sets across sectors including human and animal health, agriculture and environment at the private, local, state, national, and global levels need to be integrated to achieve rapid detection of hazards and timely response capabilities.

This issue was a common thread that emerged from all our internal and external discussions and subject matter experts we interviewed. It has been highlighted on numerous occasions when assessing past disease outbreaks and epidemics such as influenzas, West Nile virus, SARS, BSE, and food- and water-borne outbreaks, including Salmonella and E. coli.

Discussion

Private and public agencies participate in biosurveillance activities across human and animal health, agricultural, and environmental sectors. Within private and public human and animal sectors, a great deal of data is already being collected. Sharing information across sectors, however, does not always occur. Expansive biosurveillance information is scattered across the public, private, federal, state, local, academia, non-profit, and global organizations.

Collection of biosurveillance data within the private sector varies regarding what type of data is collected and at what level. Many private companies within the food and agriculture industry collect such data routinely, but the data from these sources are poorly utilized and coordinated.

In addition to the food and agriculture industry, those participating in biosurveillance activities within the private sector include laboratories, medical facilities (including human and animal hospitals and clinics), poison centers, research facilities, and universities. In many cases, similar facilities collect potential biosurveillance information in the public sector (publicly funded universities versus private universities, for example).

Global, national, state, county, and municipal governments vary widely. States' statutes and constitutions define the nature, distribution and power of local and county government. Within the US alone there are currently 3,143 counties, many of which are further subdivided into independent and self-governing municipalities. Each government can—and in many cases does—have its own biosurveillance and data collection agencies. Policy, legal, technical, fiscal control, and authorization barriers have prevented integration of key data and information, and a substantial gap will remain if these data points are not linked.

Recommendations:

- Data and information involving animal, agriculture, food, and environmental sources that might present a human health hazard must be shared, coordinated, analyzed, and synthesized across organizations, jurisdictions, agencies, and the private sector to achieve an efficient and fully integrated biosurveillance strategy.

- A National Biosurveillance staff should coordinate and facilitate this recommendation. However, the implementation and data collection still resides within respective organizations and jurisdictions. The financial and legal components needed to achieve this recommendation should be incorporated into a national strategy.

Issue #3

Many human health hazards are inherently components of larger ecological systems. These systems arise through the convergence of people, animals, and our environment. A singular focus on human health surveillance will often miss the origin, transmission processes, and maintenance sites of potential hazards. Furthermore, the detection and response to threats may be delayed resulting in more widespread and sustained outbreaks and much more costly response and control mechanisms. An effective biosurveillance strategy must be more holistic and integrated, and we should shift our monitoring and diagnostics closer to the source of the hazard or threat. Currently, many environmental surveillance systems have been limited to clean-up sites, waste handling, chemical release, and hazardous material accidents. There are also standards to promote safe water. Although these systems are very helpful, a more proactive and comprehensive risk-based, real-time environmental biosurveillance system has not been realized. Such a system needs to be incorporated into a national strategy.

Discussion

As our population continues to grow and becomes increasingly interconnected, our environment has been altered, contaminated, and stressed in unprecedented ways. This is especially apparent globally and has been accentuated by the creation of large urban and peri-urban settings and industrialization. Billions of domestic and wild animals share our environment and add to its potential hazards. The convergence of animal and environmental health with human health is creating new exposures to human health hazards and sources of microbial, chemical, and toxic contamination. Biological, chemical, and potential radiological hazards found at known sites are closely monitored, but many exposures are increasingly found at unknown locations and are broadly distributed through water and land sources. The environment represents new sources of human health hazards, and the response to and amelioration of such hazards is an increasing complex and vexing issue.

The issue is further complicated by the fact that many exposures to chemicals and toxins take place at low levels over time and may lead to cumulative effects and chronic disease conditions. Most existing surveillance systems specially focus on acute hazardous events, but biosurveillance should also consider long-term, low level exposures that represent serious health threats. This is especially problematic when we consider shrinking water resources globally.

The TF met with subject-matter experts and reviewed existing environmental databases. We discussed critical issues with the EPA and CDC experts on water-borne illnesses, poison control centers, and with agriculture and animal health experts.

Recommendations:

- Expand biosurveillance to include environmental sites of greatest threat to human health. This expansion should incorporate more microbial and chemical testing and involve more recreational and drinking water sites and systems not currently assessed. In addition, a National Biosurveillance strategy should consider low level, non-acute exposure that, over time, may result in human health hazards and chronic illnesses and conditions.
- A National Biosurveillance staff should coordinate and facilitate this work, but implementation must continue to be coordinated and facilitated by state and local environmental protection organizations and agencies including private corporations.

Issue #4

A key area of emphasis and concern with NBAS is ultimately implementation. NBAS will necessitate data sharing, systems integration, efficient and timely exchanges of information, standardized diagnostic platforms, interoperable information technologies, broad data access, and high utility of system reports and results to ensure cost-effectiveness of operations. Thus, there need to be operating principles to guide system design and execution of recommendations. This issue was discussed within the TF, and the TF reviewed lessons learned from development of other surveillance systems and personal experiences.

Discussion

Effective execution will be determined by the skill and commitment of the NBAS leadership. For NBAS to be successful, a coherent biosurveillance system must be embedded into the organization's personnel, strategies and operational plans and actions. NBAS needs to focus, at least initially, on existing systems and data sources. Resources need to be used only for the highest priority recommendations and those that are feasible, leveraged, serve the greatest need, address the greatest threats and risks and are the most cost-effective. Animal and environmental domains should not be neglected, and any operational strategy needs to assure that the surveillance systems from these domains remain a high priority in NBAS. The TF further discussed and highlighted three critical cross-cutting issues for consideration as NBAS becomes operational:

1) Designing new electronic health information systems to support NBAS needs. Health information technology is in rapid flux nationally, driven generally by the requirements of the health reform act and by health information technology investments. Of particular relevance to NBAS activities is the planned development of "meaningful use" requirements during the next several years. These requirements are intended to ensure that electronic health records will be deployed in hospitals and providers' offices to support a wide array of functions. The meaningful use criteria for public health have yet to be articulated. It will be important to ensure that the needs of all NBAS sectors are well represented in these deliberations. This is especially true for the animal and environmental health perspectives, which might not otherwise be articulated clearly.

2) Ensuring public health access to electronic health data. It will be necessary to ensure that the electronic health information that will be increasingly available is accessible to public health practitioners to support NBAS goals. Examples of issues that need to be addressed include:

- **Privacy protection.** While the Health Insurance Portability and Accountability Act (HIPAA) includes a provision for public health use of protected health information, the way in which holders of this information ("covered entities") interpret their compliance needs, for example for disclosure, can complicate ready access to this information, especially when a public health agency requires information from multiple providers. Harmonization of the requirements, for instance through development of model policies and procedures, would reduce the transaction costs for effective use of electronic health information.

- **Distinguishing between public health practice and research.** There remains considerable lack of clarity about the boundary between public health practice and research, with similar activities being classified differently in different locations or at different times. A clearly articulated standard will reduce this uncertainty.

- **Need for standardization.** The availability of electronic health information does not assure its usability for public health purposes. There is a need to develop and then update computable definitions for public health conditions of interest. The public health community will need to adopt a standards mechanism that develops and tests definitions for conditions of interest that can be applied rigorously to electronic health data. It will also be necessary to create a mechanism to keep these definitions current, as new diagnoses, tests, and treatments are adopted in clinical practice and translated from animal and environmental health systems.

- **Consolidation of requests for information.** It will be necessary to develop efficient mechanisms for public health agencies to share information from health care delivery systems and other sources including animal health systems. While data holders may be persuaded to make information available for public health purposes, they will want to be assured that the information requests adhere to fair information practices, e.g., minimum necessary data is requested; and to be able to provide information to serve multiple public health functions simultaneously. Thus, when separate public health users need certain data, it will be advantageous for them to develop a mechanism to pool their requests, so the data holders do not need to evaluate and respond to multiple requestors, some of whom will ask for similar or identical data.

3) Establishing priorities. The many valid responses to NBAS needs will almost certainly exceed available personnel and financial resources. It will thus be important to develop a framework for prioritizing the use of resources that will exist through assessment of likely health benefits that can be achieved. This analysis should take into account the probability of specific events, their potential health impact, and the potential for mitigation. This analysis should be sufficiently quantitative to guide resource allocation.

Recommendations:

- The implementation of NBAS strategies and actions will be more difficult to achieve than creating the recommendations from this report. NBAS leadership needs to create a set of operational principles to guide and inform decisions and resource allocation, setting priorities, gaining access and sharing data, considering meaningful use requirements, adopting standardization for IT and diagnostics, and ensuring both the incorporation and integration of key animal, animal product and environmental surveillance data.

Appendix II: Acknowledgements

The Subcommittee was aided in its deliberations by the testimony and advice of many knowledgeable and experienced individuals, and the efforts of a dedicated Subcommittee and staff. Consultants, Federal Liaisons, and CDC Senior Scie0tists to the Subcommittee and working groups contributed ideas and report materials.

The Subcommittee thanks the **NBAS Consultants to the Working Groups:**

Governance (Interagency Collaboration and Engagement)

Pamela Diaz, Centers for Disease Control and Prevention (CDC) – Public Health Surveillance Program Office (PHSPO)

Healthcare & Public Health Information Exchange

Laura Conn, Centers for Disease Control and Prevention (CDC) – Public Health Informatics and Technology Program Office (PHITPO); **Taha Kass-Hout,** Centers for Disease Control and Prevention (CDC) – Public Health Surveillance Program Office (PHSPO)

Innovative Information Sources

Taha Kass-Hout, Centers for Disease Control and Prevention (CDC) –Public Health Surveillance Program Office (PHSPO)

Global and Regional Biosurveillance Coordination

Ray Arthur, Centers for Disease Control and Prevention (CDC) – Division of Global Disease Detection and Emergency Response (DGDDER); **John Ridderhof,** Centers for Disease Control and Prevention (CDC) – National Center for Emerging and Zoonotic Infectious Diseases (NCEZID); **Alexandra Levitt,** Centers for Disease Control and Prevention (CDC) – Office of Infectious Diseases (OID)

Biosurveillance Workforce, New Professions & Cross-training

Denise Koo, Centers for Disease Control and Prevention (CDC) – The Scientific Education and Professional Development Program Office (SEPDPO); **Pat Drehobl,** Centers for Disease Control and Prevention (CDC) – The Scientific Education and Professional Development Program Office (SEPDPO); **Mehran Massoudi,** Centers for Disease Control and Prevention (CDC) – The Scientific Education and Professional Development Program Office (SEPDPO)

Integrated Multi-Sector Information

Carol Rubin, Centers for Disease Control and Prevention (CDC) – Division of High-Consequence Pathogens and Pathology (DHCPP)**; Colleen Martin,** Centers for Disease Control and Prevention (CDC) – Division of Environmental Hazards and Health Effects (DEHHE)**; Amy Funk-Wolkin,** Centers for Disease Control and Prevention (CDC) – Division of Environmental Hazards and Health Effects (DEHHE)**; Art Liang,** Centers for Disease Control and Prevention (CDC) – National Center for Emerging and Zoonotic Infectious Diseases (NCEZID)

The Subcommittee thanks the **Federal Liaisons in the following NBAS Working Groups:**

Governance (Interagency Collaboration and Engagement)

Teresa Quitugua, United States Department of Homeland Security

Healthcare & Public Health Information Exchange

Laura Conn, Centers for Disease Control and Prevention (CDC) – Public Health Informatics and Technology Program Office (PHITPO); **Taha Kass-Hout,** Centers for Disease Control and Prevention (CDC) – Public Health Surveillance Program Office (PHSPO)

Innovative Information Sources

David Lipman, United States Department of Health and Human Services – National Institute of Health; **Michael Kurilla,** United States Department of Health and Human Services – DMID, NIAID, NIH, Office of BioDefense Research Affairs; **Randy Kincaid,** United States Department of Defense, Defense Threat Reduction Agency

Global and Regional Biosurveillance Coordination

Raul Sotomayor, United States Department of Health and Human Services; **Capt. Clifford Brown,** United States Department of Homeland Security; **Ray Arthur,** Centers for Disease Control and Prevention (CDC) – Division of Global Disease Detection and Emergency Response (DGDDER)); **John Ridderhof,** Centers for Disease Control and Prevention (CDC) – National Center for Emerging and Zoonotic Infectious Diseases (NCEZID)

Biosurveillance Workforce, New Professions & Cross-training

Denise Koo, Centers for Disease Control and Prevention (CDC) – The Scientific Education and Professional Development Program Office (SEPDPO); **Mehran Massoudi,** Centers for Disease Control and Prevention (CDC) – The Scientific Education and Professional Development Program Office (SEPDPO)

Integrated Multi-Sector Information

Teresa Quitugua, United States Department of Homeland Security; **Jessica Pulz,** United States Department of Agriculture, Office of Homeland Security and Emergency Coordination; **Carol Rubin,** Centers for Disease Control and Prevention (CDC) – Division of High-Consequence Pathogens and Pathology (DHCPP)

The NBAS would like to thank **Dr. Thomas R. Frieden**, CDC Director for his recognition of the importance of biosurveillance and the ongoing support of the NBAS.

The Subcommittee wishes to thank **Curtis Weaver**, CDC; **Mark Byers**, CDC; **Christine Bradshaw**, CDC; **Prachi Mehta**, CDC; **Michael Latham**, CDC; **Julie Lipstein**, L3 STRATIS; **Randy Mitchell**, L3 STRATIS; **Daniel Morris**, L3 STRATIS; **Christina Zackery**, L3 STRATIS; **Richard White**, L3 STRATIS; **Stacey Smith**, McKing Consulting Corporation; **Shu McGarvey**, Northrup Grumman; **Danielle Stewart**, Lockheed Martin; **Lindsay Oweida**, Deloitte Consulting LLP; **Matthew Boulton**, University of Michigan Medical School; **Dr. Ruth Maeschiro**, AAMC; **James Tyson**, CDC; **Anthony Williams**, ChemSpider; **Kevin Russell**, GEIS; **Virginia Lee**, CDC; **David Ross**, Task Force for Global Health; **Eric Myers**, DOD; **May Chu**, CDC, **Jay Morris**, FDA; **Cynthia Lucero**, VA; **Christina Egan**, Wadsworth Center; **Larry Granger**, USDA; **Michael Beach**, CDC; Division of Public Health Surveillance and Program Office (PHSPO); **Sylvain Aldighieri** Division of Public Health Surveillance and Program Office (PHSPO), PAHO; **Roberta Andraghetti**, PAHO; **Kerri Ann Jones**, OES/IHB; **Louise Gresham**, NTI; **Matthew Hepburn**, NSS; **Richard Hatchett**, NSS; **Franca Jones**, NSS; **Toni Boni**, USAID; **Don Shriber**, CDC; **Alan Rudolph**, DTRA; **Rebecca** Daley, DOS; **Ana West**, DOS; **Scott Dowell**, Program and GDD Operations Center, CDC; **Partick Kelley**, IOM; **Ben Petro**, EOP; **Jose Fernandez**, HHS; **Phillip Lambach**, WHO; **Murray Trostle**, EPT; **Ron Yoho**, DTRA; **Dan Lowe**, BEP; **Tricia Schmitt**, OMB; **Kevin DeCock**, CDC for their hard work in supporting the meetings of the NBAS and repeated attention to the ongoing needs and support of the Subcommittee.

www.ingramcontent.com/pod-product-compliance
Lightning Source LLC
Chambersburg PA
CBHW080610290526

45790CB00007B/2714